ACHILLES TENDON SURGERY DIET

Unlocking The Power Of Nutrition And Optimizing Recovery For Reclaiming Strength And Muscle Healing

DR LUCAS KAYCE

DISCLAIMER

This book about illness and nutrition is not meant to replace expert medical advice, diagnosis, or treatment; rather, it is meant purely for informational reasons. This book's content is founded on broad concepts and recommendations for managing diseases and nutrition.

Before adopting any major dietary or lifestyle changes, readers are recommended to speak with a qualified healthcare provider, such as a licensed physician or registered dietitian, especially if they have pre-existing medical concerns. Everybody has different health demands, so what works for one person might not work for another.

The use of the information provided in this book may have unfavorable repercussions or consequences, for which the author and publisher disclaim all liability. No disease is meant to be identified, treated, cured, or prevented by the information provided.

The book may include contain references to medical literature or research findings; however readers are urged to independently confirm this material and contact reliable sources.

It is important to remember that the fields of nutrition and medicine are always changing, and that new findings could have an impact on the advice offered in this book. As a result, readers are urged to keep up with the most recent advancements in healthcare and, when in doubt, seek professional counsel.

By reading this book, readers agree that they are in charge of their own health decisions and release the author and publisher from any liability arising from the use of the material in the book, whether direct or indirect.

TABLE OF CONTENTS

ABOUT THE BOOK

The book "Achilles Tendon Surgery Diet" offers a thorough explanation of how important nutrition is to the healing process after Achilles tendon surgery. The book discusses many facets of nutrition, acknowledging the importance of a well-organized diet plan in the healing process. It provides insightful analysis and useful guidance for both the pre- and post-surgery stages.

This book explores the essential steps that must be taken to be ready for Achilles tendon surgery. It discusses the value of speaking with surgeons, providing advice on what to eat before surgery, and how to take dietary supplements to get your body in the best possible shape for a successful procedure.

An adequate diet is essential for a quick and efficient recovery following surgery. The fundamentals of postoperative nutrition are covered in this chapter, with special attention to the importance of maintaining a balanced intake of macronutrients that are essential for the healing process and drinking enough water.

This book offers a thorough analysis of foods having anti-inflammatory characteristics, with an emphasis on the role nutrition plays in lowering inflammation. It talks about using anti-inflammatory foods and spices, such as omega-3 fatty acids, to promote a more wholesome healing process.

Protein plays a crucial role in the healing process following Achilles tendon surgery. This chapter explains the function of protein in the healing process, lists high-quality protein sources, and offers suggestions for the ideal protein consumption to aid in the body's healing processes.

This book examines the function of particular vitamins and minerals in the healing process, emphasizing their significance. It discusses the importance of vitamin D, the relationship between vitamin C and collagen synthesis, and the function of minerals in preserving bone health.

A vital component of the healing process is hydration. This chapter highlights the significance of adequate hydration, exploring the nuances of electrolyte balance and offering helpful advice for preserving ideal levels of hydration during the healing process following Achilles tendon surgery.

Because practicality is essential, this chapter offers meal planning and nutrient-dense recipe ideas to help readers prepare balanced meals. With sample meal plans catered to several phases of recuperation, it provides a helpful manual for sustaining a balanced and nourishing diet.

Sustaining a healthy weight is necessary for full recuperation. This chapter examines weight-management techniques, offering advice on how to modify calorie intake and take a comprehensive approach to promote general well-being while undergoing rehabilitation.

This book discusses how nutritional considerations can be incorporated into rehabilitation since it acknowledges the connection between physical therapy and nutrition. It gives advice on how to use diet to speed up rehabilitation and on how to maintain healing over the long term.

The book explores the relationship between diet and mental health, which is frequently disregarded. It looks at how eating well can help with stress and anxiety management, emotional health, and developing a healthy connection with food during recovery.

CHAPTER ONE

ACHILLES TENDON SURGERY DIET OVERVIEW

KNOWING ABOUT SURGERY ON ACHILLES TENDONS

The strong fibrous band that connects the calf muscles to the heel bone is known as the Achilles tendon, and problems with it can be treated medically with Achilles tendon surgery.

Surgery is usually advised for those who have had severe damage or injury to the Achilles tendon, such as rips, ruptures, or long-term illnesses that compromise the integrity of the tendon. Comprehending the complexities of Achilles tendon surgery entails exploring the anatomy of the lower leg, the particular ailments that require surgery, and the range of surgical methods that physicians utilize.

The Achilles tendon is essential for the lower limbs to function properly and is important for actions like walking, running, and jumping. This tendon's injuries can have a major effect on everyday activities and mobility. When conservative measures, such as physical therapy or immobilization, fail to restore the tendon's strength and functionality, surgery is frequently recommended. The choice to have Achilles tendon surgery is a complicated one that requires careful consideration of the patient's general health, the extent of the injury, and the possible advantages and disadvantages of the operation.

DIET IS CRUCIAL TO THE HEALING PROCESS

The healing and rehabilitation period that follows Achilles tendon surgery is a crucial component of the procedure. The postoperative phase is essential to guaranteeing a favorable result and averting problems. A well-planned, nutritionally balanced diet followed by the patient is a critical component that impacts the healing process.

It is impossible to exaggerate the impact that nutrition plays in the healing process because it promotes tissue mending, lowers inflammation, and supports general health.

 Following Achilles tendon surgery, a well-balanced diet full of vital vitamins, minerals, and nutrients is crucial for encouraging tissue repair and lowering inflammation. Particularly important to the healing process are proteins, which are needed for the creation of collagen, the protein that makes up tendons' structural structure.

Maintaining tissue flexibility and facilitating the delivery of nutrients to the healing site require enough hydration. Furthermore, oxidative stress can be warded off with the support of an antioxidant-rich diet, which fosters a more favorable healing environment.

Comprehending Achilles tendon surgery necessitates a thorough examination of the intricate anatomical details and surgical methods utilized. Realizing the critical function a balanced diet plays in the healing process is equally crucial.

CHAPTER TWO

CONSULTATION WITH SURGEON

It is imperative to have a thorough consultation with the surgeon before having Achilles tendon surgery. The patient and the surgeon can talk about the procedure's specifics, possible dangers, and anticipated results during this first meeting. The surgeon will evaluate the patient's medical history, the present state of health, and any prior conditions that could affect the procedure or recuperation period during this session.

The surgeon will perform a comprehensive examination of the Achilles tendon and may use imaging tests, such as MRIs or X-rays, to assess the degree of injury. The patient can also discuss any worries, ask questions, and have a full understanding of the surgical procedure during the consultation. The surgeon could share information about the expected time frame for recovery, post-operative care, and exercises for rehabilitation. It is crucial to have open lines of communication during this session to make sure that the patient and the surgeon have the same expectations and objectives.

PREOPERATIVE DIETARY GUIDELINES

The success of any surgical treatment, including Achilles tendon surgery, is greatly dependent on good nutrition. To maximize their body's preparation for the impending operation, people should follow preoperative dietary recommendations in the weeks preceding the procedure. A diet high in nutrients and well-balanced can help with wound healing, inflammation reduction, and post-operative recuperation.

In general, doctors advise patients to concentrate on eating a diet high in proteins, vitamins, and minerals. Including complete grains, lean meats, fruits, and vegetables can help the body heal damaged tissue and strengthen its immune system. Sufficient hydration is also essential for optimum performance and recuperation. Limiting one's intake of processed meals, sugar-filled drinks, and foods heavy in saturated fats can help reduce inflammation and improve surgical results.

NUTRITIONAL SUPPLEMENTS

To promote their general health and recuperation, patients undergoing Achilles tendon surgery may want to include some nutritional supplements in addition to eating a well-balanced diet. Because of their well-known anti-inflammatory qualities, omega-3 fatty acids may help to lessen inflammation surrounding the surgery site. Vitamin C and zinc supplements are important because they aid in the production of collagen, which is necessary for tissue repair.

To maintain bone health, calcium and vitamin D supplements could also be advised, especially if any treatments relating to the health of the bones are part of the surgery. Before starting any new supplements, people should, however, speak with their healthcare professional because taking too much of some vitamins and minerals might have negative consequences.

A comprehensive strategy for getting ready for Achilles tendon surgery includes careful discussion with the physician, following preoperative dietary recommendations, and thinking about the right nutritional supplements. By attending to these elements, people can improve their general state of health, maximize their body's preparedness for surgery, and facilitate a more seamless recuperation.

CHAPTER THREE

BASICS OF POST-SURGERY NUTRITION

A SYNOPSIS OF POSTOPERATIVE NUTRITION

A vital component of the healing process, postoperative nutrition has a key role in accelerating healing, lowering complications, and improving the patient's general state of health. The postoperative phase is marked by elevated metabolic requirements and a greater requirement for nourishment to facilitate the healing of injured tissue and the immune system. Therefore, patients and healthcare workers must understand the fundamentals of postoperative nutrition.

THE VALUE OF PROPER HYDRATION

A vital component of postoperative diet, adequate hydration plays a major role in the overall efficacy of the healing process. To avoid dehydration, which can impair organ function, slow healing, and raise the risk of complications, it is essential to maintain an appropriate fluid balance.

Additionally, dehydration might make it more difficult for the body to rid itself of pollutants, impeding its normal detoxification processes. To meet the increased hydration needs during the postoperative period, patients are frequently recommended to eat enough water and, in certain situations, electrolyte-rich beverages.

MACRONUTRIENT EQUILIBRIUM

Another important aspect of postoperative nutrition is balancing macronutrients, including carbs, proteins, and lipids. Every macronutrient contributes differently to the healing process. The body uses carbohydrates as its main energy source to power its metabolic processes. Sufficient consumption of carbohydrates keeps the body from using proteins as fuel, allowing them to be used for their vital functions in immunological response and tissue repair.

Essential amino acids form proteins, which are necessary for immune system maintenance and the synthesis of new tissues.

To promote wound healing and avoid muscular atrophy, postoperative patients frequently need to consume more protein. In the meantime, fats offer a concentrated source of energy and aid in the absorption of fat-soluble vitamins.

Individualized food regimens are also essential, considering the patient's medical background, particular surgical treatment, and general state of health. Patients having gastrointestinal procedures, for example, may require dietary adjustments due to reduced nutrient absorption. In some circumstances, medical practitioners could advise taking specific dietary supplements to fill in any dietary deficiencies and encourage the best possible recovery.

Postoperative nutrition regimens place a strong emphasis on nutrient-dense foods to make sure patients get the vitamins and minerals they need to support their bodies' healing processes. Postoperative patients have a variety of dietary demands, which can be met by including a mix of fruits, vegetables, lean proteins, whole grains, and healthy fats. Furthermore, it can be advised to eat small, frequent meals to improve nutrition absorption and avoid gastrointestinal discomfort.

Postoperative nutrition is a complex and ever-changing area of medicine that needs to be handled with caution and customized strategies. A focus on nutrient-dense foods, balanced macronutrient consumption, and adequate hydration all help to optimize the healing process and promote better postoperative results. Through comprehension and use of these concepts, medical professionals and patients alike can take a proactive role in fostering a smooth recovery and restoring ideal health following surgery.

CHAPTER FOUR

LOW-INFLAMMATORY DIET

FOODS TO LOWER INFLAMMATION LEVELS

A key component of the anti-inflammatory diet, which promotes the consumption of foods recognized for their capacity to counteract inflammation in the body, is reducing inflammation through dietary choices. Many foods have been found to have anti-inflammatory qualities, therefore including them in your diet can improve your general health and wellbeing.

ADDITION OF OMEGA-3 FATTY ACIDS

Fatty seafood like sardines, mackerel, and salmon is one of the foods that is advised for lowering inflammation. Omega-3 fatty acids, especially docosahexaenoic acid (DHA) and eicosapentaenoic acid (EPA) are abundant in these fish and have been linked to anti-inflammatory properties. Consuming these fish can improve cardiovascular health and help control inflammation.

Nuts and seeds, along with fatty fish, are great providers of nutrients that reduce inflammation. Omega-3 fatty acids and antioxidants found in almonds, walnuts, flaxseeds, and chia seeds may help reduce inflammation. These foods offer a straightforward option to support an anti-inflammatory lifestyle because they are simple to add to meals, snacks, salads, and yogurt.

Fruits and vegetables are essential components of any diet that reduces inflammation. A wealth of antioxidants, vitamins, and minerals may be found in berries, cherries, leafy greens, and cruciferous vegetables like broccoli and Brussels sprouts. These nutrients help to fight inflammation and oxidative stress. These vibrant, nutrient-dense meals are essential for lowering chronic inflammation in addition to improving general health.

It's crucial to have omega-3 fatty acids in the diet to maximize its anti-inflammatory effects. These important fats are found in plant-based foods including flaxseeds, chia seeds, and hemp seeds in addition to fish. Omega-3 and omega-6 fatty acid balance can be preserved by consuming a range of these sources; an imbalance may exacerbate inflammation.

SPICES & HERBS TO REDUCE INFLAMMATION

Another essential component of the anti-inflammatory diet is herbs and spices. Anti-inflammatory and antioxidant qualities are well-known for garlic, ginger, cinnamon, and turmeric. The key ingredient in turmeric, curcumin, has been the subject of much research due to its ability to lower inflammation and possibly even help prevent chronic illnesses. These herbs and spices can enhance the flavor and health benefits of meals when added to food or added to drinks like tea.

The foundation of an anti-inflammatory diet is thoughtful food selection that gives a high priority to nutrient-dense and anti-inflammatory foods.

CHAPTER FIVE

FOODS HIGH IN PROTEIN FOR HEALING

PROTEIN'S FUNCTION IN RECUPERATION

As the basic building block of all tissues, muscles, and cells, protein is essential to the healing process. The body needs more protein to help tissue regeneration and repair after stress or injury, such as during illness, surgery, or vigorous physical activity. Amino acids, which make up protein, are necessary for the synthesis of new proteins that promote wound healing and general recuperation.

When it comes to healing, protein catalyzes several biochemical processes, encouraging the synthesis of hormones and enzymes that aid in the restoration of injured tissues.

Furthermore, protein helps the immune system by aiding in the production of immune cells and antibodies, both of which are essential for protecting the body from infections and diseases.

Throughout the healing process, a robust and resilient immune response depends on consuming an adequate amount of protein.

Moreover, collagen is a structural protein that gives tissues like skin, tendons, and ligaments strength and suppleness. Collagen is formed primarily of protein. Because it aids in the development of scar tissue and the healing of the wounded area, collagen is especially crucial to the healing process of wounds. As a result, getting enough protein is crucial to giving the body the tools it needs to rebuild and repair damaged tissues, resulting in a more rapid and efficient recovery.

SOURCES OF SUPERIOR-GRADE PROTEIN

For the best possible recovery, high-quality protein sources are crucial since they offer the full range of essential amino acids required for different body activities. Because they contain all of the essential amino acid profiles, animal-based proteins including lean meats, poultry, fish, eggs, and dairy products are regarded as high-quality sources. The complete range of necessary amino acids required for tissue repair and protein synthesis is provided by these proteins.

Legumes, nuts, seeds, and whole grains are examples of plant-based protein sources that can supplement a diet high in protein for healing. For those who only consume plant-based foods, it's crucial to make sure their consumption is varied and to combine various plant foods to get the whole spectrum of amino acids. Protein complementation is a technique that guarantees the body gets all the necessary building blocks for the best possible recovery.

Foods high in protein supply the essential amino acids as well as extra nutrients like vitamins and minerals that support general health. For example, omega-3 fatty acids, which are abundant in fish and have anti-inflammatory qualities, aid in the healing process even more. A varied and nutrient-dense diet that promotes healing can be attained by choosing meals high in protein from both plant and animal sources.

SUGGESTIONS FOR PROTEIN CONSUMPTION

The amount of protein required for healing depends on several variables, including the person's age, weight, degree of exercise, and type of injury or disease. To fulfill the increased need for tissue regeneration and immunological function during recovery, healthcare providers typically advise consuming a higher protein intake.

The Recommended Dietary Allowance (RDA) for protein for inactive adults is 0.8 grams per kilogram of body weight; however, a higher consumption may be beneficial for those in recovery.

Under certain circumstances, medical professionals might suggest consuming between 1.2 and 2.0 grams of protein per kilogram of body weight for those who are physically active, recuperating from surgery, or managing long-term medical conditions. Sufficient consumption of protein is essential not only for quick healing but also for long-term health maintenance and muscle preservation.

CHAPTER SIX

MINERALS AND VITAMINS FOR HEALING

VITAMIN C AND THE FORMATION OF COLLAGEN

When it comes to collagen formation in particular, vitamin C is essential to the body's healing process. Collagen is a type of structural protein that gives blood vessels, tendons, ligaments, and skin strength and suppleness. Because it functions as a cofactor for the enzymes involved in the creation of collagen, vitamin C is necessary for the synthesis of collagen. Sufficient quantities of vitamin C promote the robustness and integrity of connective tissues, which aid in the restoration and recuperation of tissues injured in sports or other accidents.

Apart from its function in collagen synthesis, vitamin C is a potent antioxidant. Free radicals, which are erratic chemicals that can harm cells, are countered by antioxidants. activity, particularly vigorous activity, has been shown to boost the generation of free radicals.

By scavenging these free radicals, vitamin C contributes to the overall healing process by shielding cells from oxidative stress.

THE VALUE OF VITAMIN D

Let's talk about the role that vitamin D plays in recuperation. This fat-soluble vitamin is essential for many physiological processes. The maintenance of bone health is one of vitamin D's primary roles. Vitamin D promotes mineralization and bone strength by making it easier for the intestines to absorb calcium and phosphorus. Maintaining ideal vitamin D levels is essential for bone development and regeneration during the healing process, particularly following fractures or strenuous physical activity that strains the skeletal system.

Furthermore, vitamin D has been linked to immune system regulation and muscular function. Sufficient amounts of vitamin D are necessary for healthy muscles and for the contraction of muscles, which enhances physical activity performance and lowers the risk of injury. Moreover, vitamin D contains immunomodulatory properties that support the immune system's ability to respond appropriately to obstacles, which is necessary for a quick and effective healing process.

MINERALS FOR HEALTHY BONES

Because they contribute to the density and structural integrity of bones, minerals are essential to bone health. Bone tissue is made up primarily of trace minerals, including calcium, phosphorus, magnesium, and others. For example, calcium is an essential mineral that gives bones their strength and stiffness. Getting enough calcium in your diet is essential for preventing bone-related problems and promoting bone healing following stress or injury.

Another necessary mineral that contributes to the structural makeup of bone mineralization is phosphorus. It maintains bone strength and density in concert with calcium.

Magnesium also aids in the absorption and utilization of calcium in bones through its role in bone metabolism. Osteoporosis and other disorders can result from a deficit in certain minerals, which can affect bone health.

Vitamins and minerals play a variety of roles in the healing process. The body heals from physical exertion, injury, or other challenges with the help of essential minerals that contribute to bone density, vitamin D's effects on bone health, muscle function, and immune modulation, and vitamin C's role in collagen production and antioxidant activity. To promote the best possible healing and general well-being, it is imperative to balance these nutrients with a diet rich in variety and nutrition.

CHAPTER SEVEN

HYDRATION TECHNIQUES

HYDRATION IS ESSENTIAL FOR HEALING

Hydration is crucial to the healing process because it affects several physiological processes that are necessary for healing. Maintaining proper cellular activity, removing waste products from the body, and facilitating the transportation of nutrients are all dependent on maintaining adequate hydration. The body frequently needs more fluids throughout the healing process after surgeries or traumas to promote tissue regeneration and repair. These procedures can be slowed down and complications may arise as a result of dehydration. As a result, maintaining appropriate levels of hydration is essential for a quick and successful healing process.

ELECTROLYTE EQUILIBRIUM

Electrolyte balance is very important when it comes to healing and is directly related to hydration. Electrolytes are minerals that have an electric charge and are essential for neuron activity, muscular contractions, and fluid equilibrium. Examples of these minerals are calcium, magnesium, sodium, and potassium. The body may encounter variations in electrolyte levels during the healing process, particularly if there is inflammation or an increase in activity. Sustaining the proper balance of electrolytes becomes crucial to assist the body's general healing processes. Drinking electrolyte-rich liquids and staying properly hydrated both contribute to maintaining and restoring this delicate equilibrium.

TIPS FOR STAYING HYDRATED AFTER ACHILLES TENDON SURGERY

Adopting targeted hydration measures is crucial for those recovering from Achilles tendon surgery to achieve optimal healing outcomes. The Achilles tendon is an essential part of the lower limbs, and proper postoperative care is necessary after surgery on this sensitive structure. Maintaining enough hydration is essential for promoting the body's natural healing processes because it facilitates the delivery of nutrients to the injured area and facilitates the removal of metabolic waste products. It also maintains the general health of the musculoskeletal system and helps to avoid issues like blood clots.

 A mix of drinking enough water and concentrating on electrolyte-rich fluids is recommended for hydration during the healing phase following Achilles tendon surgery. It is essential to stay hydrated throughout the day to avoid dehydration, which can impede the healing process.

Adding electrolyte-containing drinks, like coconut water or sports drinks, can also aid in restocking vital minerals that can be depleted throughout the healing process. Urine color can be used as a straightforward indicator of one's level of hydration; a pale yellow tint indicates adequate hydration.

 Incorporating foods high in water, like fruits and vegetables, will also help you stay hydrated overall. Consuming foods high in water content, such as cucumber, celery, and watermelon, helps the body retain water while supplying vitamins and minerals that aid in the healing process. To ensure a well-rounded approach to recovery that includes proper hydration and electrolyte balance, patients recovering from Achilles tendon surgery must work closely with their healthcare providers to tailor hydration strategies based on their unique needs and medical conditions.

CHAPTER EIGHT

RECIPES AND MEAL PLANNING

MAKING WELL-COMPOSED MEALS

One of the most important parts of eating a healthy, well-rounded diet is preparing balanced meals. Together with a range of micronutrients (vitamins and minerals), a balanced meal usually consists of a combination of macronutrients (proteins, fats, and carbohydrates). Giving the body the nourishment it requires for optimum performance is the aim. Including a source of lean protein, whole grains, a range of vibrant veggies, and healthy fats in each meal is a popular strategy for reaching balance. This blend guarantees a varied nutritional composition and aids in controlling energy levels all day long.

Creating balanced meals requires considering portion sizes in addition to macronutrients. Moderation is essential since imbalances can result from consuming too much of any one nutrient. Including a variety of foods from various food, categories give meals more variety and enjoyment in addition to offering a spectrum of nutrients. The taste and nutritional value of well-balanced meals can be further improved by experimenting with various cooking techniques and seasonings.

EXAMPLE MEAL SCHEDULES FOR VARIOUS REHAB STAGES

Planning meals is essential to helping people recover from a variety of conditions, including illness, surgery, and strenuous exercise. Meal plans that are customized for individual needs maximize nutrient intake and speed up the healing process. For instance, to ease the burden on the digestive system in the early phases of recuperation, foods that are readily digested may be prioritized. Soups, broths, and soft, easily chewed foods may fall under this category.

Meal plans might be modified as recuperation advances to incorporate a greater range of nutrient-dense foods to promote general healing.

A meal plan for someone recuperating after strenuous exercise can emphasize meals high in protein to support muscle regeneration and foods high in carbohydrates to restore glycogen stores. To create customized meal plans based on unique health concerns, nutritional preferences, and recovery objectives, speaking with a healthcare provider or nutritionist is necessary.

SIMPLE AND HIGH-NUTRIENT RECIPES

Making simple, high-nutrient dishes is a useful strategy for people with hectic schedules or little experience in the kitchen. A quinoa salad with an array of vibrant greens, lean protein sources like grilled chicken or chickpeas, and a tasty dressing made with olive oil and herbs is one example of this type of dish. This meal offers a variety of vitamins and minerals from the various veggies in addition to a well-balanced blend of macronutrients.

Another flexible choice is a smoothie, which is made by combining yogurt, fruits, vegetables, and a protein source like protein powder or nut butter.

This simple recipe is a great way to get your recommended daily allowance of nutrients in while having breakfast, as a snack, or even as a post-workout recovery meal. One-pan dinners that combine a variety of veggies, lean proteins, and whole grains also make cooking easier while producing a nutrient-dense, well-rounded dish.

Uncomplicated and nutrient-dense recipes, meal plans customized to various stages of recovery, and the creation of balanced meals are all crucial elements of a long-term, healthful approach to nutrition. These behaviors furnish the body with essential nutrients, facilitate recuperation, and render healthy eating pleasurable and accessible, hence augmenting general well-being.

CHAPTER NINE

CONTROLLING WEIGHT WHILE RECOVERING

SUSTAINING A HEALTHY WEIGHT

Keeping a healthy weight is essential for general well-being, particularly while recovering. Weight control must be given top priority when recuperating from surgery, a medical condition, or any other health setback to assist the body's healing processes. Immune system performance, energy levels, and overall healing results are all boosted when one maintains a balanced weight.

A person's capacity to maintain a healthy weight may occasionally be impacted by changes in appetite or metabolism that occur throughout the healing process. It is imperative to pay attention to these shifts and modify eating habits as needed.

This can entail selecting nutrient-rich snacks to maintain energy levels throughout the day or eating smaller, more frequent meals to account for changes in appetite.

STRATEGIES FOR MANAGING WEIGHT

To ensure that people can balance their dietary needs and physical health, weight management techniques are essential. The secret is to take a holistic strategy that includes regular exercise, a balanced diet, and thoughtful lifestyle decisions. Concentrating on nutrient-dense foods, such as fruits, vegetables, lean meats, and whole grains, helps the body recuperate by providing vital vitamins and minerals.

Keeping up with physical activity is still crucial to controlling weight when recovering. Exercise regimens must be customized to each person's degree of fitness and the nature of their recuperation process. Walking and mild stretching are examples of low-impact exercises that can enhance muscle tone, improve circulation, and help manage weight without putting too much strain on the body.

MODIFYING CALORIE CONSUMPTION

Changing one's calorie intake is a key strategy for managing weight while recovering. During the healing process, the body may demand different amounts of energy, thus it's important to match calorie intake to individual needs. Speaking with medical specialists, such as dietitians or nutritionists, can offer tailored advice regarding the right calorie intake depending on the kind of recovery, age, gender, and activity level.

Furthermore, practicing mindful eating can improve the success of weight management initiatives during the healing process. Maintaining a healthy weight can be facilitated by exercising portion control, being aware of when you are hungry and full, and avoiding emotional eating.

Deep breathing exercises and other relaxation-promoting activities can also assist regulate stress, which otherwise may have an impact on eating behaviors.

Controlling weight while recovering is a complex process that calls for striking a good balance between exercise, nutrition, and general well-being. A holistic approach can help people support their bodies more effectively during the healing process, which will speed up recovery and promote long-term health and vitality.

CHAPTER TEN

PARTICULAR OBSERVATIONS REGARDING REHABILITATION

DIETARY HABITS AND PHYSICAL THERAPY

In the process of recovery, nutrition is crucial, especially when combined with physical therapy. The goal of this complementary relationship between healthy eating and physical therapy is to maximize the recuperation and general well-being of patients undergoing rehabilitation. The efficiency and speed of rehabilitation can be greatly impacted by dietary factors, with special focus paid to supplying the nutrients required to promote healing and improve physical function.

DIETARY ADVICE TO HASTEN REHABILITATION

Dietary advice becomes crucial in the context of physical therapy and nutrition to expedite the healing process. For example, getting enough protein is essential because it aids in tissue regeneration and muscle restoration, both of which are critical for those recovering from operations or accidents. Lean protein sources include fish, chicken, beans, and dairy products can help maintain and grow muscle mass while a patient is undergoing rehabilitation.

Moreover, general health and recuperation depend on eating a well-balanced diet high in vitamins and minerals. Vitamin C, D, calcium, and zinc are among the nutrients that are essential for healthy bones, a strong immune system, and tissue regeneration.

To guarantee a varied and nutrient-dense diet that promotes the body's healing processes, include a range of fruits, vegetables, whole grains, and dairy products.

Another important component of diet during recovery is hydration. Maintaining proper hydration is critical for temperature regulation, nutrient movement throughout the body, and joint lubrication. Rehab patients, particularly those receiving physical therapy, should make drinking plenty of fluids a priority to maximize the benefits of their treatments and assist the body's healing processes.

EXTENDED NUTRITIONAL ASSISTANCE

Sustaining rehabilitative success requires long-term nutritional support in addition to urgent dietary considerations. To sustain the gains made throughout recovery, it is imperative to adopt healthy eating practices as a way of life. Teaching people about mindful eating, portion control, and sustainable food choices improves their general health and helps them avoid setbacks or relapses.

Professionals in physical therapy and nutrition must work together to provide a holistic approach to rehabilitation. Individualized diet regimens that are in line with needs and objectives can improve the efficacy of physical therapy treatments.

CHAPTER ELEVEN

HEALTHY EMOTIONAL AND NUTRITIONAL STATE

THE RELATIONSHIP BETWEEN MENTAL HEALTH AND DIET

The complex connection between diet and mental health is an increasingly important subject for comprehending and fostering emotional well-being. Numerous studies have demonstrated the significant influence of nutrition on mental health, emphasizing the part specific nutrients play in neurotransmitter synthesis and brain function as a whole.

Enough consumption of vital nutrients, including vitamins, minerals, and omega-3 fatty acids, is necessary to sustain the best possible mental and emotional health. A healthy diet is essential for the brain's complex functions, and mental health issues have been associated with a higher risk of nutritional deficiencies.

HANDLING TENSION AND FEAR

In today's fast-paced environment, managing stress and anxiety is a typical difficulty that nutrition plays a critical part in alleviating. Anxiety and stress can contribute to harmful eating patterns, which can worsen emotional health in a vicious cycle. Antioxidant-rich foods like fruits and vegetables can help fight the oxidative stress brought on by long-term stress, while complex carbs like whole grains help stabilize blood sugar levels, which in turn helps people feel more balanced. Probiotic-containing meals, such as yogurt and fermented foods, may also favorably affect the gut-brain axis, which may have advantages for mental health.

DEVELOPING A HEALTHFUL CONNECTION WITH FOOD

A healthy lifestyle and the development of emotional well-being depend on developing a favorable connection with food. To do this, one must practice mindfulness and awareness when it comes to eating habits and prioritize physical nourishment over severe dieting. Having a balanced relationship with food lowers the risk of eating disorders and enhances mental health in general by assisting people in keeping a positive outlook on eating. Accepting a varied and comprehensive viewpoint on nutrition is essential since it acknowledges that contentment and enjoyment are essential elements of a positive relationship with food. Encouraging people to enjoy and relish their food cultivates a positive outlook and strengthens the link between nutrition and emotional well-being.

The relationship between diet and mental health is complex and deserving of serious thought. Understanding how a balanced diet affects neurotransmitter function and cognitive functions highlights how crucial dietary decisions are to preserving emotional health.

A mindful diet can effectively promote coping with stress and anxiety by addressing the physiological effects of these challenges. Fostering a balanced and inclusive eating style is essential to developing a positive relationship with food since it promotes both physical and mental well-being. In general, improved emotional well-being and a happier, more satisfying existence can be greatly aided by comprehending and implementing these ideas into one's lifestyle.

www.ingramcontent.com/pod-product-compliance
Lightning Source LLC
Chambersburg PA
CBHW060810260726
48660CB00002B/877